Women Bodybuilding

Build A Lean Sexy Toned Curvy Body Without Getting Bulky

Table of Contents

Contents

Introduction

I've been in the gym business for 33 years, as a gym owner, personal trainer and a bodybuilding coach. During that time, I've seen some interesting things in relation to women and their bodies. In the '80s Jazzercise was all the rage. The '90's saw the advent of Tae-bo. Then with the '00's came Cross-Fit, as women slowly cottoned on to the benefits of weight training.

During those three decades, I've helped hundreds of women totally transform their bodies from frumpy to fantastic, turning couch potatoes into bodybuilding champions. By utilizing bodybuilding training strategies, these ladies have moved beyond the myths associated with women and weights to unleash dramatic physical changes all over their bodies. In this book, I will reveal the exact same techniques, diet and training that have created these hard bodies. By following this guide you will be able to revolutionize your body and your training.

Choosing to follow the bodybuilding lifestyle will make you a stronger, fitter, sexier person. But it will also instill within you vital qualities that will help you to achieve success in all areas of life . . .

- o Discipline
- o Confidence
- o Perseverance

Ok, ready to take the first step?

It's time to turn the page on your former soft self and start hardening up…

Chapter One - Starting the Journey

So, you've decided to dip your toes into the bodybuilding waters.

Yay for you!

You have managed to steer your way past the stereotypes, the myths and the raised eyebrows that may have greeted your announcement of your new passion. You are about to discover something quite astounding and profound. . .

The sport of bodybuilding brings with it a rewarding experience that can provide you with a vast array of benefits that go far beyond the sense of accomplishment that comes from winning a competition.

You will also receive amazing health benefits for your inner body – the part that others can't see. Your cardiovascular system will be functioning optimally, your bones, joints and immune system will all be stronger. And, of course, you will begin to look amazing on the outside. You'll also be strong. That means that you will be less susceptible to injury and more able to handle the demands of life. All of which makes you wonder why you didn't jump into the bodybuilding lifestyle years ago!

But wait – there's more. Bodybuilding will develop vital mental skills that will improve every area of your life. You will be focused, more goal driven, more disciplined and more able to overcome barriers to achievement.

In short, bodybuilding will make you a fitter, healthier, sexier, stronger, mentally tougher person. So, let's get started on this journey . . .

Where Are You Now?

The first step on your bodybuilding journey involves taking stock of where you're at right now. It's a bit like those pre-tests that you used to take at school. You want to find out the following:

- Your raw weight
- Your lean body mass
- Your body fat percentage
- Your key bodily measurements (chest, waist, upper arms, thighs, calves)

You will want to get hold of a good set of scales. Ideally your scales will have a built in body-fat function. If not, get yourself a set of body fat calipers and follow the instructions on how to use them. If you are planning on joining a gym, you can expect a fully body analysis and fitness test on your first session. So, whatever way you accomplish it, you will need to find your body fat percentage.

Once you have your overall weight and body-fat percentage you will be able to calculate your lean body mass. Simply multiply the overall weight by the body-fat percentage. Then subtract the fat amount from the total weight to get your lean body mass.

Here's an example:

Raw weight =65 kg

Body-fat percentage = 28%

Actual Body-fat = 18.2 kg

Lean Body Mass = 48.8 kg

Now you know exactly where you're starting from. You're in a position to monitor every ounce of muscle gain – as well as how much fat you're losing.

Next you'll need a decent tape measure with which you can take your key muscle measurements. Take the measurements around the mid part of the muscle and be as accurate as possible – every centimeter counts.

Machines or Free Weights

Machines are great for teaching beginners good form and helping them to learn what it feels like to lift correctly. That's because they ensures good form. They're also excellent for isolating individual muscles and are the way to go for those who are recovering from injury. On the other hand, machines are not as multi-functional as free weights. The frame of the machine doesn't allow for ideal exercise position for all body types. Nor does it promote functional strength. In addition, machines cannot provide anything but an approximate match between a person's strength curves and the machine's resistance curves.

Work-Out Recommendations

- Use machines for the first 6 weeks of your training in order to learn how to perform the movement
- After that, opt for free weights for your basic movements like squats, bench press and deadlifts
- Use machines and cables as secondary movements to provide isolation of the working muscle

Chapter Two - Meet Your Body

Bodybuilding is all about knowing your body and how to build, shape and refine every part of it. To do that you've got to be familiar with your muscles. In this section, we'll provide an overview of the key skeletal muscles that you will be working with, from front to back.

Front of Body

Shoulders (Deltoids): A three headed muscle that features anterior, middle and posterior portions. The shoulders are involved in every upper body movement as they perform the actions of abduction and adduction (pulling the arms away from and toward the body). The deltoids are also capable of rotation.

Chest (Pectorals): Two muscle groups comprise the chest – the pectoralis major and the pectoralis minor. These muscles perform adduction (pushing the away from the body) as well as medial rotation.

Biceps Brachii: There are two heads to the biceps, the long head and the short head. It is able to perform two function – flexion at the elbow and supination at the elbow. The Brachialis is a small muscle that runs from the ulna to the elbow. It assists with elbow flexion.

Forearm (Brachioradialis): The forearm's key function is elbow flexion.

Abdominals (Rectus Abdominis): The abdominals consist of the rectus abdominis, the external obliques and the internal obliques. The rectus abdominis is involved in flexion of the trunk. The external obliques allow for lateral flexion of the trunk as do the external obliques.

Thighs (Quadriceps): The rectus femoris runs along the mid thigh area. It performs flexion and extension. The vastus muscles run on either side of the femoris and perform extension of the leg. The adductors are situated close to the hip joint and allow for adduction, lateral rotator flexion and medial rotation.

Calves: The Gastrocnemius forms the main part of the calf muscle. It's job is to allow for flexion at the ankle. The soleus muscles run below the gastrocnemius on either side of the lower leg. It assists in ankle flexion.

Back of Body

Trapezius: The trapezius runs between the neck and the shoulders, all the way down to the lower spine. It allows for upper elevation of the scapula, as well as adduction and depression of the scapula.

Lats (Latissimus Dorsi): The lats have their origin at the lower four ribs and insert on the medial side of the humerus. This muscle provides the much sought after "V" shape to the upper body. It provides for extension, adduction and medial rotation.

Middle Back (Rhomboids): The Rhomboids have their origin at the spine and insert at the scapula. Their function is adduction of the scapula.

Lower Back (Lower Trapezius): The lower trapezius allows for depression of the scapula.

Glutes: The gluteus maximus, medius and minimus provide for extension, lateral rotation and abduction of the lower body.

Hamstrings: The hamstrings are comprised of the rectus femoris, the semitendinosus and the semimembranosus muscles. They provide for extension and flexion of the upper leg.

Chapter Three - Beginner's Training Principles

. **Specificity:** If you want to compete on the Miss Olympia stage you are going to train a whole lot differently than a house wife who's focused on firming your middle after her 3rd baby. That's the principle of specificity. A specific result requires a specific training program. You therefore, are using the weights as a tool to achieve your ends. An example of the principle of specificity in action could relate to a basketball player. The principle dictates that the exercises he chooses will mimic what he does on the court. For legs, he can choose squats or he can choose leg extensions. Squats more closely mimic the jumping movements required in basketball, whereas leg extensions are an isolation exercise. The basketball player would choose to do squats.

. **(2) Overload:** The overload principle means that you need to be constantly lifting more weight, performing more repetitions or decreasing your between set rest than you did during your last workout.

. **(3) Progressive Resistance:** This principle dates way back to Milo of Croton, a 6th century, BCE wrestler. Legend tells us that, as a boy, Milo started carrying a newborn calf every day as it grew to maturity. The calf got heavier every day, but, because the increments were so small, Milo didn't notice them. By the time the bull had grown to maturity, Milo was able to carry it around his family farm. Weight trainers have been drawing inspiration from Milo ever since. By increasing the weight by small increments each workout, you'll be able to dramatically improve your strength, which will enhance your intensity and boost your fat loss results.

. **(4) Intensity:** Intensity relates to the amount of effort you put into your training sessions. If you are working out at the optimal intensity, the last 2 or 3 repetitions of each set should be difficult to perform. If you finish a set and you feel like you could perform another 2 or 3 reps then you are not working at sufficient intensity. You need to either increase the weight, increase the reps or decrease the rest between each set.

- **(5) Rep Range:** Rep range relates to the number of times that you perform a movement. To get the most out of your training you need to ensure that you are using the ideal number of reps for your specific training goal. The traditional rep ranges are as follows: 4 to 7 reps for strength8-12 reps for building muscle 13-20 reps for fat loss and endurance

- **(6) Volume:** Volume relates to the number of sets and reps required for optimal training. This is an area of much debate, with advocates of extremely low volume training (one set per exercise) citing scientific studies to support their view just as passionately as those who swear by high volume training (20 sets per body part). The sensible approach lies somewhere in the middle. 3-4 sets per working set seems to be about ideal.

- **(7) Rest:** The period of time that you rest between sets is critical. It can range from very short (30 seconds) to very long (3 minutes +). You need enough time to recover from the last set just enough to allow for a full out effort on the next one. If you rest too long then your intensity level will stay at the same level. You want to build from one set to the next. For that reason you will rest for 60 seconds between each set.

- **(8) Tempo:** Tempo relates to the speed with which you perform your repetitions. Every rep has two distinct parts, the lifting (concentric) and the lowering (eccentric). During the concentric part of the lift, your muscle is shortening or contracting. It lengthens during the eccentric phase of the movement. It is imperative that you use a controlled tempo which allows you to isolate the working muscle and avoid momentum in the lift. An ideal training tempo is to take 2 seconds on the concentric part of the movement and 4 seconds on the eccentric part. The eccentric part of the movement actually builds muscle more than the concentric part. Doing it slower resists gravity and increases intensity.

- **(9) Variation:** Periodically changing your workout program prevents your body from becoming accustomed to the workload that is being placed upon it. This helps to avoid training plateaus and keeps your body guessing and responding. It also prevents training boredom and allows you to work your body from a variety of angles. You should change your program every six weeks.

- **(10) Recuperation:** When you work out, you are placing stress on your body. Your energy stores are depleted, your muscle tissue gets broken down and your body is put in a fatigued state. It is after the workout that recovery and rebuilding takes place. That's why you need 48 hours rest between workouts.

Chapter Four - Mentally Preparing For Your Workout

You don't want to be one of those people who just goes through the motions in the gym. They are wasting their time. Rather, take a leaf from professional athletes who treat their workouts like a battlefield mission. If you want to get the most out of your training effort, you need to apply laser like focus to every aspect of your workout. In fact, you should divide your mental training focus into 2 aspects:

Before the Workout

(1) Mentally rehearse the workout in the hour before you hit the gym. See yourself grabbing the weights and powering through those last 3 difficult reps. Focus on your immediate goal, which is to do more than you did in your last workout - an extra rep, another 2 pounds of weight or a reduced rest between sets. Do this for every exercise.

(2) Discuss your specific workout plans for that day with your buddies. Tell them you are absolutely focused on getting 8 reps with 30 pound dumbbells on the bench press. Put it out there.

(3) Surround yourself with positive people. Remember . . .*If you lay with dogs, you'll get up with fleas.*

Actively seek out people who will support you. They will pull you up when you need it and reinforce your daily goals.

(4) Be distracted early. When you first walk into the gym, pause to take in the surroundings. Check out who's there and what's different. Doing this early allows you not to be distracted when you flick the switch and your workout begins.

(5) Build up your inner drive. An hour before your workout, your engine should be idling at a 4. By the time you walk into the gym it should be up to a 7. During your warm-up, it's reached 8.5. And by the time you pile the weight on for your first set, you're hitting 10.

During the Workout

(1) Focus directly on the working muscle group. Get connected. If you are doing barbell curls, put your mind into your biceps. Let nothing else matter. That way you'll be able to fully engage a muscle and recruit as many muscle fibers as possible.

(2) Switch off your brain. At least the part of it that is bent on sabotaging your workout. You know the part. It's constantly trying to rationalize with you to get you to do less. So you don't injure yourself. So you don't run out of time. So you don't over-train. Don't negotiate with this side of your brain. Instead, tell your brain that what you're doing is easy. Don't focus on the weight that you're lifting. Visualize your body as a machine, your arms and legs as pistons, mechanically driving the weight up and down.

Chapter Five - The Ultimate Nutrition Guide

What you eat is more important than how you train. Unfortunately, the world at large has made this subject so confusing that most people throw up their hands in frustration and resort to what they've always been doing. In this section we will make it easy to follow a sound nutritional plan that will allow you to provide the perfect anabolic environment to support your bodybuilding efforts. It will be built upon 4 principles:

(1) Eat Frequently
(2) Balance Your Macronutrients
(3) Avoid Refined Carbs and Sugar
(4) Drink Water

Let's take them one at a time:

Eat Frequently

Do you ever skip breakfast, not eat anything until noon, and then complain that you can't get any results from your exercise? Or do you eat a perfect diet for a few days in a row and then let your diet go to hell for the next few days? You have to give your body the fuel when it needs it if you want it to perform. Eating your entire day's allotment of calories in one pig-like sitting isn't going to cut it. There's a lot of evidence to suggest that our bodies will only assimilate a certain amount of calories per sitting. Any excess will be stored as fat.

Research also indicates that if you feed your body balanced meals that contain quality protein and carbohydrates throughout the day - as many as six small meals spaced out every three hours - you'll enjoy a number of spectacular benefits, including:

(1) enhanced metabolism
(2) less stomach discomfort
(3) stable energy levels throughout the day
(4) controlled appetite
(5) it provides enhanced energy for your workouts
(6) it supports muscle growth

Balance Your Macronutrients

Sensible eating requires taking in a healthy balance of protein, carbohydrate and fat. Contrary to recent media reports, carbs are not your enemy. They are, in fact, your body's preferred source of energy. You'll need them to fuel your workouts. Protein requirements for weight trainers are higher also. Those who regularly engage in weight training exercise are routinely breaking down muscle tissue. They need extra protein to repair all of this damage. What's more, they need it at specific intervals. In fact, timing of protein is very important. We need it straight after a workout, about 30 minutes later when muscle protein synthesis is at it's highest - and even before bedtime to control cortisol levels and ensure that we've got a plentiful supply of amino acids coursing through our bloodstream while we're sleeping. To meet all of your body's protein demands, aim for 1 gram of protein per pound of lean bodyweight.

Avoid Refined Carbs & Sugar

Concentrate on eating natural, unprocessed carbs. Reduce processed refined carbs as much as possible. Cut out white sugar and flour completely. Include a mixture of both starchy carbs and fibrous carbs on your plate. Eat fruit every day. Aim to take in 50% of your daily calories from carbs, with 30% coming from lean protein sources and 20% from healthy fats.

Here are a dozen refined carb and sugar laden foods to avoid like the plague:

(1)   French fries and other deep fried foods
(2)   Ice cream and milkshakes
(3)   Doughnuts and pastries
(4)   Sweets and confections
(5)   Sugar sweetened soft drinks
(6)   Sugar sweetened juice drink and energy drinks.
(7)   White bread and flour products
(8)   Crisps
(9)   Bacon, sausage and processed meats
(10)   Hot dogs and fast-food burgers
(11)   Thick crust pizza
(12)   Sugary breakfast cereals

And here are a dozen healthy foods to replace them with:

(1)   Fresh fruit
(2)   Fibrous vegetables
(3)   Yams
(4)   Potatoes
(5)   Unsweetened oats
(6)   Brown rice
(7)   Beans and pulses
(8)   100% whole wheat or whole grains
(9)   Low or fat-free dairy products
(10)   Chicken and turkey breast
(11)   Eggs and egg whites
(12)   Lean cuts of red meat

Drink Water

No one wants to be told to drink more water. It's too easy - and cheap. Everyone's looking for some super supplement that will strip away the fat at lightning speed, allowing them to reveal a ripped, shredded, fat free body to startled onlookers. To them there's only one worthwhile piece of advice -

Drink more water!

Without it nothing in your body works properly. With it everything in your body works optimally. If you ever find yourself dragging your way through a workout, it's probably because you're dehydrated. When you lose just 5% of water weight, your strength level can drop by as much as 30%. And thirst is not a good measure of hydration. So carry a water bottle with you all the time. Sip from it regularly - especially if you suddenly develop a between meal food craving. Shoot for 2.5 liters of water per day.

Peak Performance Nutrition

What follows is a sample nutritional program that will allow you to customize your own nutritional plan. It will give you guidance on how much to eat of what, when and why.

The Foundation: It's imperative that you calculate your personal nutritional needs. This calculation will initially be based upon your lean body mass (LBM). Your LBM is the best indicator of your basal metabolic needs (how many calories you need each day to function). By adding your physical activity output, we get a pretty good picture of your overall nutrient needs. This calculation will give us a good jumping of point.

Calculating your LBM: Get your body fat (BF) measured. You can either do this at your local gym, step on a pair of scales that automatically calculates BF or investing in a set of calipers and doing it yourself. To work out the amount of fat you are carrying around in pounds, multiply your weight in pounds by the percentage of BF.

213 pounds with a BF of 29% = 62 pounds of fat

Now subtract your fat pounds from your overall weight to get your LBM

213 minus 62 = 153 pounds LBM

Assess your basal caloric needs: Multiply your LBM by 12.

153 x 12 = 1836

You now need to work out your daily caloric expenditure by activity. The handiest way to do this is via the internet. There is a great site here that lists virtually every activity known.

http://www.healthstatus.com/calculate/cbc

Pop in the minutes that you engage in that activity and it will calculate the calories that each activity burns. If your activities differ throughout the week, enter each activity for the entire week and divide by 7 to get a daily average.
Now simply add your basal caloric needs to your activity needs to get your overall daily maintenance calorie requirement.

To lose fat you should reduce your maintenance level by 500 calories per day.

Protein: You should consume 1 gram per pound of LBM. There are 4 grams of protein per calorie.

Fat: Try to hit a level of 0.3 grams per pound of LBM per day. Attempt to get most of this as unsaturated, essential fats (especially from fish, flax, hemp, etc). There are 9 grams of fat pr calorie.

Carbohydrate: Carbs will be the mainstay of your performance nutrition plan. They will provide you with the high octane fuel to keep you cranking day in day out. Your overall carb intake should equal the remainder of your calorie needs after protein and fats are accounted for. There are 4 grams of carbohydrate per calorie.

Protein = 153 x 1 = 153 grams

Daily Protein Calories = 153 x 4 = 612

Fats = 153 x 0.3 = 46 grams

Daily Fat Calories = 46 x 9 = 414

Carbohydrates = Maintenance Level (say 2500 calories*) - 1026 (fat calories + protein calories) = 1474 calories

Carbohydrate = 1474 divided by 4 = 369 grams

Use this calculation to set up you nutritional plan for the first week. This will be an assessment period. Be sure to weight yourself and note your body fat percentage at the beginning and again at the end of the week. If you haven't lost 1-2 pounds, reduce by an extra 250 calories per day.

The Plan

Now that you have your nutrient foundation worked out, it's time to put in the particulars. The following schedule assumes that you work out in the afternoon.

Sample Meal:
Nutrition shake mixed with 2 cups of fresh squeezed (orange, apple, grape-fruit, peach, pear or pineapple) juice
300 mls water

Breakfast

When: 7:00 am

What: Calories; 25% of daily total; Protein 20% of daily total; Fat 30% of daily total

Why: While you'll actually be eating 6 small meals throughout the day, breakfast should include 25% of your daily calories because your body is coming off an 8-10 hour sleep. Because of that your body is in an extreme catabolic state upon waking. This solid dose of calories will go a long way toward reversing that process.

Sample Meal:

Nutrition shake
1 slice whole wheat toast with one tablespoon all-natural peanut butter and one table-spoon all-fruit jam
1/2 large grapefruit

Mid Morning Snack

When: 10:00 am

What: Calories; 10% of daily total; Protein 10% of daily total; Fat 10% of daily total; Carbs 10% of daily total.

Why: The main goal here is to top off your glycogen stores, maintain consistent blood sugar levels and continue to feed your muscles the building blocks they need as the anabolic phase of your day begins. It's best to focus on low Glycemic Index carbs here, as the fat intake is fairly low and the carbs are pretty high.

Lunch

When: 1:00 pm

What: Calories; 20% of daily total; Protein; 20% of daily total; Fat; 20% of daily total: Carbs; 20% of daily total

Why: This is a crucial meal. It can make or break your afternoon workout. If you go too heavy on the carbs, you can be wallowing in the depths of blood sugar depression by 5pm. If you go too heavy on the fats and protein, your system may still be working hard on digesting the food as you start exercising, robbing your muscles of vital blood supply and energy. Focus on water rich veggies and fruits and lean protein. This is also a good time to load up on water. It will help your food digest quickly and keep you well hydrated for your upcoming workout.

Sample Meal:

1 (3 oz grilled chicken breast)
1 medium sweet potato
2 cups steamed veggies
2 teaspoons butter
1 large pear
300 mls water

Pre-Workout Snack

When: 3:30 pm

What: Calories; 5% of daily total; Protein; 5% of daily total; Fat; 5% of daily total

Why: Nutrition sets the foundation for your workout. It is the fuel that will power you through your training sessions. Yet, there is a widespread belief out there that you shouldn't eat before you train. That, though, is the biggest mistake you can make in your training preparation - especially if you are intent on building muscle. You simply must provide your muscles with the right environment to operate at their peak.

Sample Meal
1/2 tuna sandwich with non-fat mayo
Medium apple

Post-Workout Snack

Within 45 minutes after your workout

What: Calories; 20%; Protein 20%; Fat; 10%; Carbs; 30%

Why: This is possibly the most important meal of your day. Within the 60 minutes following your workout your muscles are like sponges, waiting to soak up carbs and to replace spent glycogen stores. If you pump in carbs and protein in about a four to one ratio directly after exercise, you can not only significantly enhance glycogen replacement, but stimulate immediate muscle recuperation as well. This snack can literally flip you from catabolic to anabolic in a matter of minutes. To facilitate this process, lots of water is necessary.

Sample Meal:
 1/2 protein bar (eat the other half during your workout)

Dinner

When: Between 30 minutes after your post snack workout and one hour prior to bed.

What: Calories; 20%; Protein; 30%; Fat 20%; Carbohydrates 10%

Why: You have already hit your glycogen replacement hard in your post workout snack, and you'll be priming it again in the morning and through lunch the next day. You don't need to hit it while you're sleeping. By keeping the carbs low here and cranking up the protein and good fats, we set up a hormonal environment in the body that allows for optimal recuperation to take place while not risking fat storage. In other words you get your energy and muscle minus the fat. This is another key hydration time. Pounding 250 mls or so in the evening will help digest and utilize the proteins and keep you hydrated overnight.

Sample Meal:
 6 oz grilled salmon steak
 1/2 cup Basmati rice
 10 steamed asparagus spears
 200 mls water

Note: The above nutritional plan will definitely give you an advantage over those who are swayed by every new fad diet like waves on the ocean. Initially it will be a chore to follow this plan, what with all the percentages that you need to adhere to. Stick with it. Before long you'll know your portions without having to think about it. That's what you want. Remember this is your new lifestyle eating plan. If it takes a month to ease into it, so what? You've got the whole rest of your life to reap the benefits.

One last word - every week, allow yourself one cheat meal. Make it a lunch and eat whatever you want. Drink water though and make sure that it's just that one meal.

Nutrition Checklist

- Eat every 3 waking hours for a total of 5-6 meals per day
- Eat a sensible balance of carbohydrates, proteins and healthy fats
- Stay away from refined carbs and sugar
- Drink 2.5 liters of water per day
- Calculate your daily caloric needs
- Work out your macronutrient ratios (calories, grams) for each meal
- Eat 25% of your day's calories for breakfast
- Fuel your training with a pre-workout meal
- Within an hour of your training get quality carbs into your system
- Take in just 10% of your daily carbs for dinner
- Allow yourself a single cheat meal every week

Smart Supplementation

Why Supplement?

The right supplements - taken at the right times - can help propel you to your bodybuilding and strength training goals by doing three things. They can increase your anabolic drive, improve your workload capacity and decrease your recovery time. Individually these factors can make a big difference. Put together they will work synergistically to power you towards your goals. Let's consider them one at a time:

Anabolic Drive

The word 'anabolic' refers to the body's ability to produce more muscle tissue. Anabolic drive involves the natural production of testosterone, growth hormone (GH), insulin-like growth factor-1 (IGF-1), insulin, thyroid, cortisol and other hormones and growth factors involved in muscle growth. For athletes, it refers to the body's ability to increase its anabolic (or muscle producing) response to exercise, nutrition, supplements and other factors.

In the case of supplements, those targeted towards increasing the production of testosterone, growth hormone and insulin, and decreasing cortisol, will result in both anabolic and anti-catabolic effects, thus maximizing the anabolic drive.

Workload Capacity

Endurance or workload capacity involves your ability to maintain high quality training throughout a workout. If your capacity is limited and you don't have the energy, endurance or concentration necessary to train hard from the beginning of your workout to the end, it won't matter how well you manage the other components - nutrition, supplementation and rest. Your diet may be excellent. You may even be training properly six days a week, but if you don't have the overall energy and muscle endurance for a productive workout, you aren't going to experience maximal progress or muscle growth.

Recovery

This involves your ability to recover properly between sets as well as workouts. The goal is to ensure that the body recovers fully from the stimulus of exercise and to reduce the amount of time necessary for it to take place. Recovery is critical to muscle growth. Your body must recuperate from the catabolic process before productive protein synthesis can occur. The sooner you recover from a workout, the sooner your body can begin to respond to it and adapt by adding muscle.

When you don't recover from workouts, you can go into a state of chronic over training. You'll actually begin to lose muscle instead of gaining it. In the gym, you'll find yourself lacking the energy to do further sets at maximum ability. Even if you do manage to get through a workout without losing effort, your body still won't respond with the kind of adaptation you want - more muscle.

Certain supplements can have a strong effect on lowering recovery time and increasing muscle growth. Supplements targeting recovery can also help you handle additional stress in your training. If you want to extend workouts from four to six days a week, supplements can help you accelerate recovery to make those workouts productive. Similarly, if you're training for another sport, in addition to your bodybuilding and strength training endeavors, supplements might just spell the difference between being able to train for both effectively and having the dual training sabotage your progress in both areas.

Anti-catabolism

You can decrease the breakdown of muscle tissue both during and after exercise and thus provide potent anti-catabolic effects in several ways. A lot of substances and methods decrease muscle breakdown and have anti-catabolic effects; for example taking in adequate carbohydrates is known to have a protein sparing effect.

Certain supplements can also create an anti-catabolic effect. Cortisol is a necessary hormone and in plays a significant role in decreasing muscle stiffness and inflammation. Without normal and somewhat elevated cortisol levels, we couldn't even exercise properly - so it wouldn't matter what training, diet, drug or nutritional supplement regimen you followed. Yet, chronically elevated levels of cortisol have a catabolic effect on muscle and decreases the effect of anabolic hormones. Decreasing the amount of cortisol after exercise can provide you with an added anabolic boost by decreasing muscle tissue breakdown and increasing amnio-acid influx and utilization by muscle cells. In addition, decreasing catabolism by using appropriate methods and supplements can dramatically increase protein synthesis and muscle mass.

Substances that decrease catabolism can have anabolic effects on muscle. But like growth hormone stimulation, many nutritional supplements can also have anti-catabolic effects. Increasing dietary calories and protein and using branch chain amino acids, glutamine, alanine and other amino acids, Vitamin C, beta-carotene and other anti-oxidant vitamins have been shown to lessen muscle breakdown.

Supplements can also be used to increase insulin, Growth Hormone, IGF-1 and testosterone levels, and decrease cortisol levels and decrease cortisol levels and other anti-catabolic factors at specific times to maximize increases in lean body mass.

Smart Supplementing: Pre-Workout

- Have a meal 60 - 90 minutes before the workout
- Focus on fast release proteins and slow release carbs
- Take no fat in your pre-workout meal
- Take in 20 grams of protein and 30-40 grams of carbs
- If you are taking a pre-workout shake have it 30 minutes before the workout
- Your pre-workout shake should be whey protein based
- Take an apple with your shake
- If on a fat cutting diet, ditch the pre-workout carbs

Smart Supplementing: Post-Workout

- Take a fast acting whey protein powder shake within 20 minutes after your workout to fast track amino acids to those hungry muscle cells.
- Add 5 mls of creatine to your shake. Creatine is the most effective supplement you can use for boosting muscle size and strength.

Chapter Six - The Ideal Beginner's Routine

This program involves a handful of core exercises which will form the basis of your routine. These are multi-joint, compound exercises that require a lot of calories and that work a number of muscle groups together. They are the best exercises to get you lean. A unique feature of this program is that it involves alternating between two different workouts every training day. On Day One you do Workout A for your Upper Body and on Day Two you do Workout A for your lower body. The next session you do Workout B for your Upper Body. Not only does this keep your workouts fresh and interesting, you are also able to train your muscles from a variety of angles. This enables you to maximally stimulate the muscle fibers and bring out complete definition. By constantly switching workouts you are also able to keep your body guessing, avoid plateaus and keep moving forward.

Keep in mind that you will work out with weights 3 times per week, not four. That means that your schedule will follow this pattern:

Mon	Wed	Fri
Upper Workout A	Lower Workout A	Upper Workout B
Lower Workout B	Upper Workout A	Lower Workout A
Upper Workout B	Lower Workout B	Upper Workout A

The program uses a two day split routine. The body is divided into an upper body day and a lower body day. You train the abs every 2nd workout.
Here are the four workouts that you will perform.

Upper Body Workout A

Decline Dumbbell Row: 4 sets / 8-10 reps
Chin Ups: 3 sets / 8-12 reps
Barbell Bench Press: 4 sets / 4-8 reps
Dumbbell Incline Press: 3 sets / 8-12 reps

Dumbbell Lateral Raise: 3 sets / 8-12 reps
Dumbbell Shoulder Press: 3 sets / 4-8 reps
Lying Tricep Extension: 3 sets / 8-12 reps
Standing Supinated Dumbbell Curls: 3 sets / 8-12 reps

Lower Body Workout A

Barbell Squat: 4 sets / 4-8 reps
Farmer's Walk: 3 sets / 12 reps
Dead-lift: 4 sets / 8-12 reps
Lying Leg Curl: 3 sets / 8-12 reps
Standing Calf Raise: 3 sets / 12 reps
Hanging Leg Raise: 3 sets / 10-15 reps
Reverse Crunch: 3 sets / 15-20 reps
Plank: 1 set of 60 seconds

Upper Body Workout B

Decline Dumbbell Row: 3 sets / 8-12 reps, 1 set 20 reps
Lat Pulldowns: 3 sets / 8-12 reps
Barbell Bench Press: 3 sets / 8-12 reps
Incline Dumbbell Flyes: 3 sets / 8-12 reps
Dumbbell Shoulder Press: 3 sets / 8-12 reps
Side Lateral Raises: 3 sets / 8-12 reps
Tricep Push-down: 3 sets / 8-12 reps
Incline Dumbbell Curls: 3 sets / 8-12 reps

Lower Body Workout B

Barbell Squat: 3 sets / 8-12 reps, 1 set 20 reps
Leg Press: 3 sets / 8-12 reps, 1 set 20 reps
Lying Leg Curl: 3 sets / 8-12 reps
Standing Calf Raise: 3 sets / 15-20 reps
Kneeling Cable Crunch: 3 sets / 15-20 reps
Prone Superman: 3 sets / 15-20 reps
Side Plank: 3 sets of 60 seconds

A Note on Resistance

Selecting the appropriate weight for each exercise will require a little bit of trial and error. For the first two weeks of the program your focus should be on training your body in correct exercise technique and performance. The resistance, therefore, can be a little lighter than optimum until you are in the groove of the movement. For compound exercises such as squats, dead-lifts and bench presses you can start with just an Olympic bar. Movements that isolate the smaller muscles groups (such as lateral raises and flyes) don't require that much weight to be effective. After a couple of weeks, apply the guidelines already providing on choosing resistance (i.e. the last 2-3 reps should be the most you could do at that weight).

UPPER BODY: Workout A

Exercise 1 : Decline Dumbbell Row

Prime Mover: Latissimus dorsi, center and lower trapezius

This exercise is a modification of the standard bent over barbell row. It allows you to optimally work the large muscles of your back while minimizing the stress on your lower spine that is an inherent part of the barbell version of the exercise.

Begin by adjusting an incline bench to a low angle, about 20 or 30 degrees. If your gym doesn't have an adjustable bench, use a regular flat bench and put the rear legs up on a block. Make sure the bench is stable before beginning the exercise.

Lean over the high end of the bench so you're supporting yourself on your abdominals. To start with, the dumbbells should be slightly in front of you at about a 45 degree angle (like airplane wings). Grip them, palms facing back. Bend your elbows enough so that your shoulder blades travel out as far as they will go. The idea here is to ensure maximum range of motion for your lats and your middle / lower traps.

When you're in the correct position, you will feel a stretch across your middle back as well as in your lats.

Pull the weights up and back with the lift coming from your lats and traps, not your arms or shoulders. Concentrate on starting the movement by bringing your shoulder blades together and away from your head. As you pull, raise your chest slightly off the bench, but keep your abdominals firmly pressed against the bench to keep the pressure off your lower back. Rotate your wrists so that your palms end up facing one another. Keep your elbows close to your sides. Lift until your elbows are at waist level.

It's important that you mentally pull back and not just up. The combination of starting with the weights in front of you and pulling back activates the lower lats and ensures development of this difficult to reach area.

If you feel like you are doing a curl, you are doing this exercise incorrectly. Except for your grip, your forearms and biceps should be as relaxed as possible. Feel for the tension in your lower lats and center back. That's the key.

Next step: Reverse the motion to lower the weights. The dumbbells should end up not quite as far forward as they started, and not touching the ground. As you lower the weight, rotate your wrists so the dumbbells return to their initial 45 degree angles to the edge of the bench. Keep your elbows bent so you get the maximum stretch across the center back and in the lower abs. Remember to lean against the bench throughout the exercise to keep the strain off your lower back.

Exercise 1: Chin Ups

Prime Mover: Latissimus dorsi

Grab a chinning bar with an underhand, shoulder width grip, and hang with your elbows slightly bent. Pull your chin up above the bar, hold for a second or two, and lower your body with control. Let you legs hang straight down and don't jerk your way up. Just pull yourself up in a smooth motion and then let your body down under control.

For maximum stretch and contraction, lower yourself to the very bottom of each rep and pull up until your chin touches or goes above the bar.

If you are unable to perform one complete repetition on a chinning bar, start by doing reverse push ups. Perform reverse push ups as follows:

Fix a bar 1 meter above the ground (you can do this on a Smith machine). Lie down so that the bar is directly over your chest. Grab the bar with an overhand grip that's slightly wider than shoulder width. Lift your torso and legs off the floor so that only the back of your heels remain planted on the floor. Pull in your abs and hold your body in a straight line from head to heels.

Exercise 2: Barbell Bench Press

Prime Mover: Pectorals

Load the appropriate weight onto the bar. Lie on the bench and take a grip just wide enough so your forearms are not quite parallel. Too narrow a grip shifts the load onto the triceps and makes it difficult to feel the tension in the chest. Now pinch your shoulder blades together. Lower the bar to sternum level. Your elbows should end up at a 70 degree angle to your sides and your forearms should be vertical. Touch your chest (never bounce), forcefully stretch your pecs and immediately drive upwards, squeezing your lats and arcing the bar up to its start position at mid chest. Lock out briefly between reps. Keep your shoulders down throughout the movement.

Breathing: Inhale while the bar is overhead, hold your breath during the descent and breathe as your press back.

Exercise 3: Dumbbell Incline Press

Prime Mover: Pectorals

If the incline bench you are using is adjustable, set it to a 30 degree angle. Sit on the bench with a dumbbell in each hand. Rest the dumbbells on your thighs close to your knees. Kick up your legs, one at a time, to assist getting the weights into position up at your shoulders.

Press the dumbbells up, using your pecs to pull them up and across your chest. Keep your back flat against the bench as you lift. At the top of the movement, squeeze the pecs tightly and hunch your shoulders forward. Don't touch the weight together at the top of the exercise - keep them 2-3 inches apart. Slowly lower the weight down as far as you can, getting the greatest stretch possible.

Exercise 4: Dumbbell Lateral Raise

Prime Mover: Deltoids

Grasp a light pair of dumbbells with a closed, neutral grip. Stand with feet shoulder width apart. Hold the dumbbells out from the sides of your thighs with your palms facing inwards. Slightly flex your elbows and hold them in that position throughout the movement.

Now lift the dumbbells up and out to the sides with your hands, forearms, elbows and upper arms rising together. Do not shrug your shoulders to lift the weights. Keeping your body erect with your knees slightly flexed and feet flat on the floor, bring the dumbbells back to the starting position.

Exercise 5: Dumbbell Shoulder Press

Prime Mover: Deltoids

Sit on a bench and grasp a pair of dumbbells with a closed, pronated grip. Your head should be up and your upper back and hips should be pressed against the back pad of the seat. Move the dumbbells to position them at shoulder level with your palms facing forward. The dumbbell handles should be in line with each other and parallel to the floor.

Push the dumbbells up until your elbows are fully extended. Keep your wrists straight and directly above your elbows. Make sure, too, that you maintain your erect position. Do not lean back or lift off the bench as you press the dumbbells overhead.

Now lower the dumbbells back to the start position. Keep your wrists straight and directly above your elbows.

Exercise 6: Lying Tricep Extension

Prime Mover: Triceps

Lie on a flat bench with a barbell across your thighs. Position yourself so that the base of your head is against the end of the bench (in other words, so most of your head is off the bench). Grab the barbell with a narrow, palm down grip and kick your legs back to get the bar into position above your head. Your arms should not be straight up and down. Rather, they should be inclined slightly backward and toward the head. This angle keeps tension on the triceps throughout the entire exercise. Bend your knees and hook your feet against the end of the bench.

Starting in this position, lower the bar to your forehead, keeping your forearms parallel to each other and your upper arms stationary. Don't allow the elbows to drift apart. Non-parallel forearms greatly decrease the effectiveness of the exercise and increase the strain on your elbows.

Press the bar back up to the inclined position. Concentrate on keeping your upper arms parallel.

Exercise 7: Standing Supinated Dumbbell Curls

Prime Mover: Biceps

Begin with a dumbbell in each hand, palms facing forward. You can increase your stability and decrease general strain during this exercise by performing this movement leaning against a bench with your knees slightly bent. Think of the exercise as a combination of two movements that must be smoothly integrated.

The first is supination of the forearm. This involves rotating your forearm so that your palm , which begins facing backward, ends up facing forward.

Second is a curl. Proper curling is not obvious, nor is it what the body does naturally if given a chance. The natural tendency with any exercise is to do as little work as possible. When doing curls, for example, your body adjusts to the position of greatest mechanical advantage, taking as much strain off your biceps as possible - not at all what you want to get lean, fat free upper arms.

To maximize the work done by the biceps during any curl you need to:

(1)   Make sure that your elbow and arm remain in the ideal plane throughout the movement (perpendicular to your body). You don't want your elbows to move away from the body.

(2)   Keep your elbow slightly in front of you during the curl. The natural tendency is to let the elbow move next to the body - or worse yet, behind the body - as you raise the weight. This takes the strain off the biceps.

When performing a supinated curl, both the supination of the forearm and the curling motion should occur simultaneously. The supination should not happen all at once. Try to rotate the forearm smoothly throughout the entire curling motion. A common error is to do the entire supination at the beginning of the movement. Remember to bring your elbow slightly forward as you do the curl - not back, or to the side. Keeping your elbow in front of you ensures maximum action of the long head of the bicep, which flexes the shoulder as well as the elbow.

Lean into the curl t the top of the movement to keep the tension on the biceps. On the way down it's important to exactly reverse the movement performed on the way up. Don't let your elbows drift from their position slightly in front of you. Much of the benefit of any exercise come from returning to the start position. You throw the benefit away if your form is sloppy when lowering the weight.

LOWER BODY: Workout A

Exercise 1: Squats

Prime Mover: Quadriceps

Place an Olympic bar on the squat rack. At a weight of 45 lbs you won't need to add any added weight but make sure that use a pad in the middle of the bar to protect your neck.

Position yourself under the bar and lift it off the rack. Step back and stand with your feet spread slightly wider than shoulder width and pointing slightly outward. Keep your back straight, your chest thrust out and your head up. Now tense your abdominal wall, bend your knees and lower your body until your thighs are parallel with the floor. To avoid excess strain on the knees, don't go down any further. While squatting, keep your head up and your back slightly arched.

In the bottom squat position, your lower legs should be almost vertical to the floor. Push through your heels as you return to the starting position.

Because squats include an aerobic component, it's vital that you use proper breathing technique. If you don't you may start to feel light headed after a few repetitions. As you lower yourself breathe in deeply. Then on the way back up forcefully expel the air in one breath. During the final few repetitions, take two or three quick breaths between reps.

SQUATTING NO NO'S

*** Squatting over a bench. Every time you touch the bench with your glutes, your spine will compress slightly. Over time this may cause vertebral damage.

*** Placing a block under your heels / turning your toes too widely outwards. Both of these will place unnatural stresses on your knees and, over time, can lead to injury.

*** Leaning too far forward. Not only does this increase your likelihood of suffering spinal injuries, it also takes the stress off the quadriceps and onto the trunk extensor muscles.

*** Allowing the knees to ride over the toes while allowing your heels to lift off the floor. Keeping your lower legs almost vertical may feel unnatural at first but it can make the difference between injured and healthy knees. Keeping your shin bones vertical drastically reduces your risk of injury.

Exercise 2: Farmer's Walk

Prime Mover: Quadriceps

Select a pair of light dumbbells (2 - 5 lbs) and place them in front of you in an area that allows you at least 9 feet of clearance straight ahead. Stand between the dumbbells and bend down to grip the handles. Lift the dumbbells by driving up through your heels while keeping your back straight and your head up. Take an exaggerated step that requires you to lunge. The longer the step the more emphasis is placed on your gluteus while shorter steps maximize the effect on the thighs. Pushing off with you forward leg, continue lunge walking until you have covered the set distance.

On this exercise, you'll perform 3 sets of 12 reps, lunging with both legs for a single repetition.

Exercise 3: Dead-lift

Prime Mover: Upper Back

Load a barbell and set it on the floor. Squat in front of it with your feet shoulder width apart. Grab it overhead with your hands just outside your legs, your shoulders over or just behind the bar, your arms straight and your back flat or slightly arched.

Simple as it sounds, all you really do is stand up. The key is to push with your heels and pull the weight to your body as you stand. Pause with the weight, but don't lean back, then slowly return to the starting position. Pause with the weight on the floor and reset your body over the bar. You defeat the purpose of the dead-lift if you use momentum to knock out the reps.

Exercise 4: Lying Leg Curl

Prime Mover; Hamstrings

Lie on the leg curl machine, hooking your feet under the leg curl bar. Drop your chest down flat against the bench, but keep your head up and your back arched slightly (you will be in the "Sphinx" position). Curl the bar up as high as it will go. If you can't get it up all the way, decrease the weight. Leg curls are only effective when done with correct form. It's the tension in the hamstrings that counts, not the weight.

Exercise 5: Standing Calf Raise

Prime Mover: Soleus

Position yourself under a standing calf rise machine, with your shoulders resting on the shoulder pads. Place your toes on the edge of the foot plate and stand to an upright position. Keeping your knees locked throughout the movement, raise up on your toes to fully extend your calves. Hold at the top position for a slow count of three. Now, without bending your knees, lower to stretch your calves downward.

Exercise 6: Reverse Crunch

Prime Mover: Lower Abdominals

Lie with your arms at your sides. Hold your legs off the floor with your knees bent at a 90 degree angle so that your thighs point straight up and your lower legs point straight ahead, parallel to the floor.

Crunch your pelvis towards your rib cage. Your tail bone should rise 2 to 3 inches off the floor as your knees move towards your chin. Pause, then slowly return to the starting position.

Exercise 7: Plank

Prime Over: Upper Abdominals

Get into a modified push up position with your weight on your forearms and toes. Your body should form a straight line from head to heels (don't let your back sag). Pull you abs in as far as you can, and hold this position for 60 seconds, breathing steadily. If you can't get to 60 seconds in one go, break it up into 3 sets of 20 seconds and work up to the 60 second goal.

UPPER BODY: Workout B

New Exercises

Exercise 1: Lat Pull-Downs

Prime Mover: Latissimus dorsi

Take a wide grip on a lat pull-down bar with a false overhand grip (thumb on the same side as your fingers). Keep your arms straight and your torso upright or leaning slightly back. Pull your shoulder blades together to bring the weight down. At the same time stick your chest out. Pull the bar to meet your chest. Pause with the bar 1 to 2 inches off your chest, then slowly let it rise to the starting position. Keep your chest out throughout the movement.

Exercise 2: Incline Dumbbell Flyes

Prime Mover: Upper pectorals

Lie on a bench that is inclined to 30 degrees. Hold a pair of dumbbells in an overhand grip over your mid-pec region, with your arms straight up. Make sure that your feet are firmly planted on the floor. Maintaining a slight bend in you elbows, lower the dumbbells down and back until your upper arms are parallel to the floor and in line with your ears. Then use your chest to pull the weights back up to the starting position, retracing the same route in reverse. Keep your shoulder blades pinched back towards each other throughout, and flex your pecs at the top of the movement.

Exercise 3: Side Lateral Raises

Prime Mover: Deltoids

Hold two dumbbells, one in each hand, at your sides, palms facing your sides. Your feet should be shoulder width apart with your knees slightly bent. Tense your core as you raise the weights to shoulder level (no higher). While you are lifting the weights out to the side, pretend that, instead of dumbbells, you have pitchers of water in your hands and that you are going to water some plants up at shoulder level.

Allow your elbows to bend and your forearms to drift slightly forward. As you reach the top of the movement, rotate your shoulders forward so that the front plates of the dumbbells are slightly lower than the rear plates - just as if you were pouring water. This will cause you to raise your elbows slightly. The rotation needs to come from your shoulders, not your wrists or arms.

The pouring motion positions the lateral deltoid to take the brunt of the strain. If you don't 'pour', the front deltoid helps out too much, decreasing the efficiency of the exercise.

Exercise 4: Tricep Pushdown

Prime Mover: Triceps

Stand a foot or so away from the pulley on a tricep pushdown machine, holding the bar so that the cable angles slightly away from you. Your triceps are strongest about two thirds of the way through the movement, and starting in this position adjusts the resistance curve to more closely match the triceps' strength curve.

Press the bar down in as wide a semi-circle as possible. Don't let your elbows drift back. This shortens the path the bar travels and decreases the amount of work done, limiting the effectiveness of the exercise.

As you press, keep your wrists straight and your shoulders down. Allowing the wrists to bend back increases the tendency to push straight down on the bar, instead of pressing it in a semi-circle. At the bottom of the motion, your elbows should be one or two inches in front of you, and your forearms should be parallel.

Reverse the motion to raise the bar. Allow the bar to come up until it's even with your chin.

Exercise 5: Incline Dumbbell Curls

Prime Mover: Biceps

Set an incline bar at a 75 degree angle. Grasp two dumbbells with an underhand grip, straight down at arm's length. Curl the weights towards your shoulders. Stop and squeeze when the dumbbells are 6 to 8 inches in front of your shoulders. Hold the contraction, squeezing tight, for 2 seconds. Now, slowly return the dumbbells to the starting position. Be sure to resist gravity during the negative part of the movement.

LOWER BODY: Workout B

New Exercises

Exercise 1: Leg Press

Prime Mover: Quadriceps

Sit back in the leg press station with your back against the pad and your feet shoulder width apart on the foot plate. Adjust the seat so that your knees are bent slightly more than 90 degrees. Now push the weight until your knees are straight but not locked. Keep your back flat and your neck straight. Pause, then return to the start position. Do not allow your knees to buckle inward throughout this movement. Make sure to also avoid the temptation to place your hands on your knees to help push the weight. Keep your hands firmly gripping the handles throughout the movement. You should also focus your energy into your heels rather than the balls of your feet.

Exercise 2: Kneeling Cable Crunch

Prime Mover: Rectus abdominis

Attach a rope handle to a high pulley on a cable machine. Face the machine, grab the rope and kneel in front of the weight stack. Hold the ropes at the sides of your face with your elbows pointing straight down to the floor.

Crunch your rib cage towards your pelvis without moving any other part of your lower body from its original position. Pause when your elbows approach your knees, then slowly return to the starting position.

Exercise 3: Prone Superman

Prime Mover: Erector Spinae

Lie face down with your legs straight and your arms stretched straight in front of you, with your hands on the floor. Lift your arms, head, chest and lower legs off the floor simultaneously. Hold this position for 5 seconds, keeping your head and neck at the same height as your shoulders, throughout the movement. Return to the starting position.

Exercise 4: Side Plank

Prime Mover: Obliques

Lie on your non-dominant side (if you're right handed, lie on your left side). Support your weight with that forearm and the outside edge of that foot. Your body should form a straight line from head to ankles.

Pull your abs in as far as you can, and hold this position for 60 seconds. If you can't get to 60 seconds in one go, break it up into 3 sets of 20 seconds and work up to the 60 second goal.

Repeat on the other side.

Chapter Seven - The Next Step: Customization

The above program will move you from beginner to seasoned weight trainer. Use it during the first 12 weeks of your training. By the end of those 3 months you will have totally transformed your physique. You will also become a lot stronger and your cardiovascular fitness level will soar. You will also have built and delineated the outer muscles of your body.

You will now be ready to take your training to the next level.
The key difference in your program will be that, rather than training the body in two halves (upper and lower) you will be training just two body-parts in a single workout, apart from legs which will involved 3 body-parts. The following combinations work well together:

Chest and Triceps
Back and Biceps
Thighs, Hamstrings and Calves

Intermediate Training Tips:

- Always work the largest muscle group first (chest, back, thighs)
- You should spend about 20 minutes training the large muscle group (3-4 exercises, 2-3 sets of each)
- You should spend about 15 minutes training the smaller body-part (2-3 exercises, 2-3 sets each)
- Vary your rep range between 4 and 12
- Keep your rest between sets at about one minute
- Drink water and / or a protein shake with added creatine during the workout
- Train each body-part twice per week, ensuring that you leave 48 hours between each session.
- Make compound exercises (Squats, Deadlifts, Bench Press, Bent Over Rows) the foundation of your training.
- Use dumbbells as much as possible to promote balanced development and to recruit stabilizer muscles.

From now on you will change your routine every 6 weeks. By following the principles presented in this book, you will be able to design your own training programs designed to get you closer and closer to that ideal physique.

Chapter Eight - Final Word

Within your grasp you now have all of the knowledge that you need to transform your body, taking charge of your physique and allowing yourself to wear it proudly anywhere, anytime.

Knowledge, of course, is vital. But, in itself it is never enough. Unless you actually get off the couch and start implementing what you've learnt, then you have simply wasted your time. You will never regret the decision to DO bodybuilding. Let this book mark a turning point in your life. Allow the knowledge that you now have to spur you to action, so that you begin to immediately implement the training and nutrition know-how that you have at your disposal.

Your new body is waiting for you – get out there and claim it!

Sage Surefire

Subscribe to our list to get notified of new book releases from Sage Surefire. We notify you of new book releases, updates to the books, and when a book is given away free.

http://eepurl.com/bronjj

You'll like my other books.

CrossFit Training: Build a lean, athletic, sexy body with fresh and exciting crossfit workouts

http://www.amazon.com/gp/product/B00Z14BENW?*Version*=1&*entries*=0

HIIT Workouts: Get HIIT fit, fast-track your way to a shredded, super-fit new you

http://www.amazon.com/gp/product/B010MSYK96?*Version*=1&*entries*=0

Building Muscle: Bullshit free secrets to building muscle

http://www.amazon.com/gp/product/B010INJBPS?*Version*=1&*entries*=0

www.ingramcontent.com/pod-product-compliance
Lightning Source LLC
Chambersburg PA
CBHW070352300526
45791CB00025B/2063